STOMACH ULCER COOKBOOK FOR VEGETARIAN

An easy guide with Healthy, Delicious and Plant-based Recipes to nourish your stomach and restore digestive wellness

Dr. Mary D. Torres

TABLE OF CONTENT

HOW TO USE THIS COOKBOOK

1. **Familiarize yourself with the Content:** Start by reading through the introductory sections of the cookbook to understand the principles behind the plant-based diet for stomach ulcer management. Pay close attention to the information provided on understanding stomach ulcers, their causes, symptoms, and the importance of a vegetarian diet in promoting digestive wellness.

2. **Plan Your Meals:** Take time to go through the recipe sections and make note of the dishes that appeal to you. Consider your dietary preferences, any specific ingredients you have on hand, and the nutritional value of each recipe. Plan your meals for the week, incorporating a variety of options from breakfasts, lunches, soups, salads, beverages, and desserts to ensure a balanced and satisfying diet.

3. **Prepare Ingredients and Cooking Equipment:** Before diving into cooking, ensure you have all the necessary ingredients and cooking equipment on hand. Take note of any special preparation methods or cooking techniques required for certain recipes. Preparing ingredients in advance, such as chopping vegetables or soaking grains, can help streamline the cooking process and make meal preparation more efficient.

4. **Follow Recipes Carefully:** When cooking, follow the recipes in the cookbook closely, paying attention to ingredient quantities, cooking times, and preparation methods. Be mindful of any specific instructions provided, such as simmering times for soups or blending techniques for smoothies. Adjust seasoning and flavors according to your taste preferences, but aim to stay true to the overall nutritional composition of the dish.

5. **Enjoy and Listen to Your Body:** Once your meal is prepared, take time to savor each bite and pay attention to how your body responds. Notice any changes in your digestion, energy levels, or overall well-being. Keep track of which recipes you particularly enjoy and which ones best support your digestive health. Remember that adopting a plant-based diet is a journey, so be patient with yourself and allow room for experimentation and adaptation along the way.

INTRODUCTION

Digestive health is a cornerstone of overall well-being, and the food we choose to consume plays a pivotal role in nurturing or hindering our gastrointestinal system. A plant-based diet, rich in fruits, vegetables, whole grains, and legumes, offers a multitude of benefits for individuals seeking relief from stomach ulcers.

This cookbook is designed to be your guidance on the journey to digestive wellness through nourishing yourself with a plant-based diet. Cherishing a vegetarian lifestyle can be a powerful and transformative choice, especially when faced with the challenges of stomach ulcers.

The recipes in this cookbook are carefully crafted to not only satisfy your taste buds but also to promote healing from within. Plant-based ingredients bring a myriad of essential nutrients, antioxidants, and anti-inflammatory properties that can help soothe irritated stomach linings and support the overall healing process.

Through these pages, you will discover the art of creating meals that will not only tantalize your palate but will also contribute to the restoration of your digestive balance. Every recipe is thoughtfully curated to provide you with a diverse range of flavors, textures, and nutrients, ensuring that your plant-based to soothe your stomach journey is not only healing but also enjoyable.

CHAPTER 1: Understanding Stomach Ulcer

Definition of Stomach Ulcer

Stomach ulcers can also be called peptic ulcers, it's an open sores that develop on the inner lining of the stomach. These ulcers can also occur in the upper part of the small intestine and are collectively referred to as peptic ulcers. Stomach ulcers typically result from an imbalance between the digestive fluids in the stomach and the protective mucus that covers the stomach lining.

Causes of Stomach Ulcer

Stomach ulcers which is also known as peptic ulcers can develop due to various factors. Some of the common causes include:

Helicobacter pylori (H. pylori) Infection: This bacterium is a primary cause of stomach ulcers. It weakens the protective mucous lining of the stomach and duodenum, making them more susceptible to damage from stomach acids.

Nonsteroidal Anti-Inflammatory Drugs (NSAIDs): Prolonged use of NSAIDs, such as aspirin, ibuprofen, and naproxen, can irritate and erode the stomach lining, often lead to the formation of ulcers.

Excessive Stomach Acid Production: These conditions cause an overproduction of stomach acid, such as Zollinger-Ellison syndrome which can contribute to the development of ulcers.

Smoking: Smoking increases the risk of stomach ulcers and can affect the healing process. It also contributes to other digestive issues.

Alcohol Consumption: Too much alcohol intake can irritate and erode the stomach lining which increase the risk of developing ulcers.

Stress: While stress is not a direct cause of ulcers, it can accelerate existing ulcers and delay the healing process.

Genetic Factors: Some people may have a genetic predisposition to developing stomach ulcers.

Age and Gender: Stomach ulcers can occur at any age, but older adults are more prone. Men are generally at a higher risk than women.

Common Symptoms of Ulcer

Stomach ulcers can exhibit various symptoms. The severity and nature of symptoms can vary from one person to another. However, common symptoms include:

Burning Sensation: If you are having burning or gnawing pain in the stomach, often between meals or during the night, this is a classic symptom of a stomach ulcer.

Abdominal Pain: The pain associated with stomach ulcers can be felt in the upper abdomen, it is usually below the breastbone. It may come and go, often last for minutes to hours.

Indigestion: Consistence indigestion or discomfort after eating may indicate the presence of a stomach ulcer.

Bloating: Some individuals with stomach ulcers may experience bloating, a feeling of fullness, or discomfort.

Nausea: Nausea, with or without vomiting, can be a symptom of a stomach ulcer. Vomiting may contain blood if the ulcer is bleeding.

Unexplained Weight Loss: Stomach ulcers can lead to a decrease in appetite, which can result in unintended weight loss.

Dark Stools: In cases of bleeding ulcers, the stool may appear dark or tarry due to the presence of blood.

Vomiting Blood: Severe ulcers may lead to vomiting blood, which requires urgent medical attention.

Fatigue: Chronic blood loss from a stomach ulcer can lead to anemia, causing fatigue and weakness.

Treatment of stomach ulcer

The treatment of a stomach ulcer involves a combination of lifestyle changes, medications, and, in some cases, addressing the underlying causes. Here are common approaches to treating stomach ulcers:

Medications:

Proton Pump Inhibitors (PPIs): These drugs such as omeprazole and lansoprazole, reduce stomach acid production, promoting ulcer healing.

H2 Blockers: Medications like ranitidine and famotidine also help decrease stomach acid production.

Antibiotics:

If the ulcer is caused by Helicobacter pylori (H. pylori) infection, a course of antibiotics is prescribed to eliminate the bacteria.

Antacids:

Over-the-counter antacids can provide temporary relief by neutralizing stomach acid, but they are not a long-term solution.

Cytoprotective Agents:

Medications like sucralfate help protect the lining of the stomach and duodenum, promoting healing.

Lifestyle Changes:

Diet Modification: Avoiding spicy foods, acidic foods, and caffeine can help reduce irritation. Embracing a diet rich in fruits, vegetables, and whole grains is often recommended.

Quit Smoking: Smoking can hinder the healing process, so quitting is beneficial.

Quit or Limit Alcohol Intake: Quitting or Moderating alcohol consumption is advisable to reduce irritation of the stomach lining.

Stress Management: Techniques such as relaxation exercises and mindfulness can help manage stress, which can impact ulcer symptoms.

Follow-Up Endoscopy:

In some cases, a follow-up endoscopy may be recommended to assess the healing progress of the ulcer.

Surgery (In Severe Cases):

Surgical intervention is rare but may be considered for ulcers that do not respond to medication, or in cases of complications like perforation or bleeding.

CHAPTER 2: Basics of a Vegetarian Diet for Stomach Health

Who is a vegetarian?

A vegetarian is an individual who specifically follows diets that primarily consists of plant-based foods and desist from the consumption of meat and, in many cases, other animal products. The reasons for adopting a vegetarian lifestyle can vary and may include ethical, environmental, health, or cultural considerations.

However, there are different categories of vegetarianism, each specifying the extent to which animal products are excluded:

Lacto-Ovo Vegetarian: This type of vegetarians consumes plant-based foods, as well as dairy products (lacto) and eggs (ovo), but excludes meat, poultry, and fish.

Lacto Vegetarian: Lacto vegetarians consume plant-based foods and dairy products but avoid eggs, meat, poultry, and fish.

Ovo Vegetarian: They consumes plant-based foods and eggs but avoids dairy products, meat, poultry, and fish.

Vegan: Vegans excludes all animal products, including meat, dairy, eggs, and sometimes even honey, and relies solely on plant-based foods.

Key Nutrients for Ulcer Healing

Healing from stomach ulcers involves paying attention to key nutrients that promote the repair and maintenance of the digestive system. For context, some essential nutrients that play a crucial role in ulcer healing:

Protein:

Importance: Protein is essential for tissue repair and maintaining the integrity of the stomach lining.

Sources: Beans, lentils, tofu, nuts, seeds, dairy products, and plant-based protein sources.

Vitamin C:

Importance: It aids in the formation of collagen, a protein crucial for wound healing.

Sources: Citrus fruits (oranges, lemons), strawberries, bell peppers, kiwi, and broccoli.

Zinc:

Importance: It supports the immune system and helps with tissue repair.

Sources: Legumes, seeds (pumpkin seeds), nuts, whole grains, and zinc-fortified foods.

Vitamin A:

Importance: It helps promotes tissue repair and enhances the immune system.

Sources: Sweet potatoes, carrots, spinach, kale, and other dark leafy greens.

Vitamin E:

Importance: This acts as an antioxidant that protects cells from damage during the healing process.

Sources: Nuts, seeds, spinach, broccoli, and vegetable oils.

Omega-3 Fatty Acids:

Importance: Possess anti-inflammatory properties, aiding in the reduction of inflammation.

Sources: Flaxseeds, chia seeds, walnuts, hemp seeds, and fatty fish (for non-vegetarian options).

Fiber:

Importance: Supports digestive health and helps maintain regular bowel movements.

Sources: Whole grains, fruits, vegetables, legumes, and nuts.

Probiotics:

Importance: It supports a healthy balance of gut bacteria, promoting overall digestive wellness.

Sources: Fermented foods like yogurt, kefir, sauerkraut, and kimchi.

Iron:

Importance: Iron is essential for the formation of hemoglobin, especially important if there is bleeding from the ulcer.

Sources: Lentils, beans, tofu, spinach, fortified cereals, and seeds.

B Vitamins (B6, B12, Folate):

Importance: This Play a role in cell division, DNA synthesis, and overall cellular function.

Sources: Whole grains, leafy greens, legumes, nuts, and fortified plant-based foods.

Vegetarian Food to Include

For a vegetarian diet that supports stomach ulcer healing, it's very vital to include a variety of nutrient-rich foods that are gentle on the digestive system. Some vegetarian foods to include are:

Whole Grains:

Examples: Quinoa, brown rice, oats, whole wheat bread.

Benefits: It provide fiber for digestive health and essential nutrients.

Legumes:

Examples: Lentils, chickpeas, black beans, and other pulses.

Benefits: Excellent sources of protein, fiber, and various vitamins and minerals.

Tofu and Tempeh:

Benefits: Plant-based protein sources that is versatile and easy to digest.

Fruits:

Examples: Apples, bananas, melons, berries, and pears.

Benefits: Provide vitamins, antioxidants, and natural sugars without causing excessive acidity.

Vegetables:

Examples: Leafy greens (spinach, kale), carrots, zucchini, sweet potatoes, and broccoli.

Benefits: Rich in vitamins, minerals, and antioxidants; easy on the stomach.

Nuts and Seeds:

Examples: Almonds, walnuts, chia seeds, flaxseeds.

Benefits: Healthy fats, protein, and essential nutrients.

Dairy or Dairy Alternatives:

Examples: Yogurt, kefir, or lactose-free alternatives.

Benefits: Provide calcium and protein without excessive fat content.

Healthy Fats:

Examples: Avocado, olive oil, and nuts (in moderation).

Benefits: It helps supply essential fatty acids without causing irritation.

Herbs and Spices:

Examples: Ginger, turmeric, fennel, and parsley.

Benefits: They are known for their anti-inflammatory properties and potential to soothe the digestive tract.

Fermented Foods:

Examples: Yogurt, kefir, sauerkraut, and kimchi.

Benefits: Contain probiotics that promote a healthy balance of gut bacteria.

Papaya and Pineapple:

Benefits: Contain enzymes (papain and bromelain) that may aid digestion and reduce inflammation.

Cooked Vegetables:

Benefits: Steamed or boiled vegetables are gentler on the stomach while maintaining nutrient content.

Vegetarian Food to Avoid

For individuals with stomach ulcers, there are certain vegetarian foods that may trigger symptoms or irritate the stomach lining. It's essential to be mindful of these potential triggers. These are some foods that ulcer patients may consider avoiding:

Spicy Foods:

Examples: Hot peppers, chili, and spicy sauces.

Reason: Spicy foods can increase stomach acid production and irritate the stomach lining.

Citrus Fruits:

Examples: Oranges, lemons, grapefruits, and tomatoes.

Reason: High acidity in citrus fruits can be irritating to the stomach.

High-Fat Dairy:

Examples: Full-fat milk, cheese, and creamy desserts.

Reason: High-fat foods may stimulate acid production and slow down the healing process.

Coffee and Caffeinated Beverages:

Examples: Coffee, tea, and certain sodas.

Reason: Caffeine can increase stomach acid production and contribute to irritation.

Chocolate:

Reason: Contains compounds that may relax the lower esophageal sphincter, allowing stomach acid to flow back into the esophagus.

Alcohol:

Examples: Beer, wine, and spirits.

Reason: Alcohol can irritate the stomach lining and increase acid production.

Carbonated Beverages:

Examples: Soda, sparkling water.

Reason: Carbonation can lead to bloating and increase pressure in the stomach.

Fried and Greasy Foods:

Examples: Fried snacks, french fries, and deep-fried foods.

Reason: High-fat and greasy foods can be difficult to digest and may exacerbate symptoms.

Peppermint and Spearmint:

Reason: Mint can relax the muscles that separate the stomach from the esophagus, potentially leading to acid reflux.

Raw Garlic and Onions:

Reason: Both can be strong irritants to the stomach lining.

Sour Pickles and Vinegar:

Reason: High acidity in pickles and vinegar can be harsh on the stomach.

Highly Processed and Spicy Vegetarian Alternatives:

Examples: Spicy vegetarian sausages, highly processed meat alternatives.

Reason: These may contain additives and spices that can be irritating.

Importance of a Vegetarian Diet for Healing

Adopting a vegetarian diet can be of significant importance for individuals seeking healing, especially for conditions like stomach ulcers. Reasons why a vegetarian diet is beneficial for the healing process:

Reduced Acidic Load:

Plant-based diets tend to be naturally lower in acidity compared to diets high in animal products. This can help reduce the overall acidic load on the stomach, potentially minimizing irritation to ulcerated areas.

Anti-Inflammatory Properties:

Many plant-based foods, such as fruits, vegetables, nuts, and seeds, are rich in anti-inflammatory compounds. These can contribute to the reduction of inflammation in the digestive tract which promotes a healing environment.

High Fiber Content:

Vegetarian diets are typically rich in fiber from fruits, vegetables, whole grains, and legumes. Adequate fiber intake supports regular bowel movements and helps maintain a healthy digestive system.

Nutrient-Dense Foods:

Plant-based diets offer a wide array of essential nutrients, including vitamins, minerals, antioxidants, and phytochemicals. These nutrients play crucial roles in tissue repair, immune function, and overall well-being.

Improved Gut Microbiota:

The consumption of plant-based foods, particularly those high in fiber promotes a diverse and healthy gut microbiota. A balanced and thriving microbiome is associated with improved digestion and immune function.

Lower Saturated Fat Intake:

Vegetarian diets often have lower saturated fat content compared to diets rich in animal products. Limiting saturated fats can contribute to cardiovascular health and overall well-being.

Weight Management:

Plant-based diets may support weight management, which is important for individuals with stomach ulcers. Maintaining a healthy weight can reduce the risk of complications and promote general health.

Potential Reduction in H. pylori Impact:

Some studies suggest that a vegetarian diet may have a positive impact on Helicobacter pylori (H. pylori) infection, a common cause of stomach ulcers. Plant-based compounds may have antimicrobial properties that could aid in managing this infection.

CHAPTER 3: Breakfast Bliss to Start the Day

1. Banana and Almond Butter Overnight Oats

Benefits:

Gentle on the stomach with no acidic ingredients.

Bananas offer natural sweetness and potassium.

Almond butter adds healthy fats and protein.

Ingredients:

1/2 cup rolled oats

1/2 cup almond milk, 1 ripe banana, mashed

1 tablespoon almond butter

1 teaspoon chia seeds

Preparation:

In a jar, combine rolled oats, almond milk, mashed banana, almond butter, and chia seeds.

Mix well, cover, and refrigerate overnight.

In the morning, stir and enjoy cold or warm.

Nutritional Value:

Fiber: 8g

Protein: 7g

Calories: 300

Preparation Time: 5 minutes (plus chilling time)

2. Spinach and Mushroom Tofu Scramble

Benefits:

Tofu provides plant-based protein.

Spinach offers vitamins and minerals.

Mushrooms add flavor without acidity.

Ingredients:

1/2 cup firm tofu, crumbled

1 cup spinach leaves, chopped

1/2 cup mushrooms, sliced

1 clove garlic, minced

1 tablespoon olive oil

Salt and pepper to taste

Preparation:

Sauté garlic in olive oil until fragrant.

Add crumbled tofu, spinach, and mushrooms. Cook until tofu is golden and vegetables are tender.

Season with salt and pepper.

Nutritional Value:

Fiber: 5g

Protein: 12g

Calories: 250

Cooking Time: 10 minutes

3. Blueberry Chia Seed Pudding

Benefits:

Chia seeds provide omega-3 fatty acids.

Blueberries offer antioxidants and vitamins.

Ingredients:

3 tablespoons chia seeds

1 cup almond milk, 1/2 cup fresh blueberries

1 teaspoon honey (optional)

Preparation:

Mix chia seeds and almond milk in a jar.

Stir well, cover, and refrigerate for at least 2 hours or overnight.

Top with fresh blueberries and drizzle with honey if desired.

Nutritional Value:

Fiber: 8g

Protein: 5g

Calories: 220

Preparation Time: 5 minutes (plus chilling time)

4. Avocado and Tomato Toast on Whole Grain Bread

Benefits:

Avocado provides healthy fats.

Tomatoes offer vitamins and freshness.

Whole grain bread is gentle on the stomach.

Ingredients:

2 slices whole grain bread

1/2 avocado, sliced

1 medium tomato, sliced

Salt and pepper to taste

Preparation:

Toast whole grain bread slices.

Layer sliced avocado and tomatoes on top.

Season with salt and pepper to taste awesome.

Nutritional Value:

Fiber: 6g

Protein: 8g

Calories: 280

Preparation Time: 5 minutes

5. Mango and Pineapple Smoothie Bowl

Benefits:

Mango and pineapple provide vitamins A and C.

Smoothie bowls offer hydration and nutrients.

Ingredients:

1 ripe mango, peeled and diced

1/2 cup pineapple chunks

1/2 cup almond milk

1 tablespoon shredded coconut

2 tablespoons granola

Preparation:

Blend mango, pineapple, and almond milk until smooth.

Pour into a bowl and top with shredded coconut and granola.

Nutritional Value:

Fiber: 6g

Protein: 4g

Calories: 250

Cooking Time: 5 minutes

6. Cucumber and Mint Infused Water

Benefits:

Hydration is crucial for overall well-being.

Cucumber and mint provide refreshing flavor without acidity.

Ingredients:

1/2 cucumber, thinly sliced

5-6 fresh mint leaves

1 liter water

Preparation:

Combine cucumber slices and mint leaves in a pitcher.

Add water and refrigerate for at least 2 hours.

Nutritional Value:

Hydration is essential for overall health.

7. Chickpea and Vegetable Breakfast Wrap

Benefits:

Chickpeas offer protein and fiber.

Vegetables provide essential nutrients.

Whole grain wraps are gentle on the stomach.

Ingredients:

1 whole grain tortilla

1/2 cup canned chickpeas, drained and rinsed

1/4 cup bell peppers, diced

2 tablespoons hummus

Fresh spinach leaves

Preparation:

In a bowl, mix chickpeas, bell peppers, and hummus.

Warm the tortilla and spread the chickpea mixture on it.

Add fresh spinach leaves and wrap.

Nutritional Value:

Fiber: 7g

Protein: 10g

Calories: 280

Preparation Time: 10 minutes

8. Pumpkin and Chia Seed Muffins

Benefits:

Pumpkin is easy on the stomach and rich in vitamins.

Chia seeds provide omega-3 fatty acids.

Ingredients:

1 cup canned pumpkin puree

2 tablespoons chia seeds

1 cup almond flour

2 eggs

Preparation:

Mix pumpkin, chia seeds, almond flour, and eggs.

Pour into muffin cups and bake at 350°F (175°C) for 20 minutes.

Nutritional Value:

Fiber: 6g

Protein: 8g

Calories: 230

Cooking Time: 20 minutes

9. Coconut Yogurt Parfait with Berries

Benefits:

Coconut yogurt provides probiotics for gut health.

Berries offer antioxidants and vitamins.

Ingredients:

1 cup coconut yogurt

1/2 cup mixed berries (strawberries, blueberries)

2 tablespoons granola

1 tablespoon honey

Preparation:

In a glass, layer coconut yogurt, mixed berries, and granola.

Drizzle with honey.

Nutritional Value:

Fiber: 5g

Protein: 7g

Calories: 220

Preparation Time: 5 minutes

10. Cauliflower Hash Browns with Avocado Mash

Benefits:

Cauliflower is a low-calorie, cruciferous vegetable.

Avocado adds healthy fats and creaminess.

Ingredients:

2 cups grated cauliflower

1/2 avocado, mashed, 1 tablespoon olive oil

1/2 teaspoon garlic powder

Salt and pepper to taste

Preparation:

Mix grated cauliflower with garlic powder, salt, and pepper.

Form into patties and cook in olive oil until golden brown.

Mash avocado and spread on top of the cauliflower hash browns.

Nutritional Value:

Fiber: 5g

Protein: 8g

Calories: 180

Cooking Time: 15 minutes

11. Papaya and Kiwi Smoothie

Benefits:

Papaya and kiwi provide digestive enzymes.

Smoothie is easy on the stomach and hydrating.

Ingredients:

1 cup papaya, diced

1 kiwi, peeled and sliced

1/2 cup Greek yogurt

1/2 cup coconut water

1 tablespoon honey

Preparation:

Blend papaya, kiwi, Greek yogurt, and coconut water until smooth.

Sweeten with honey to taste.

Nutritional Value:

Fiber: 5g

Protein: 6g

Calories: 200

Cooking Time: 5 minutes

12. Vegetarian Breakfast Burrito

Benefits:

Eggs provide protein.

Vegetables offer essential nutrients.

Whole grain tortilla is gentle on the stomach.

Ingredients:

1 whole grain tortilla

2 eggs, scrambled

1/4 cup black beans, cooked

1/4 cup salsa

Fresh cilantro, chopped

Preparation:

Scramble eggs and cook until fluffy.

Warm the tortilla, layer with eggs, black beans, salsa, and cilantro.

Roll into a burrito.

Nutritional Value:

Fiber: 6g

Protein: 15g

Calories: 320

Preparation Time: 10 minutes

13. Zucchini and Tomato Frittata

Benefits:

Zucchini is gentle on the stomach.

Tomatoes add flavor without acidity.

Eggs provide protein.

Ingredients:

1 zucchini, sliced

1 cup cherry tomatoes, halved

4 eggs

1/4 cup feta cheese, crumbled

Salt and pepper to taste

Preparation:

Sauté zucchini in a pan until slightly softened.

Add cherry tomatoes and cook for a few minutes.

Whisk eggs, pour over vegetables, and sprinkle with feta.

Bake at 350°F (175°C) until set.

Nutritional Value:

Fiber: 4g

Protein: 14g

Calories: 280

Cooking Time: 25 minutes

14. Chia Seed and Berry Parfait

Benefits:

Chia seeds offer omega-3 fatty acids.

Berries provide antioxidants and vitamins.

Ingredients:

3 tablespoons chia seeds

1 cup almond milk

1/2 cup mixed berries (strawberries, blueberries)

2 tablespoons sliced almonds

1 tablespoon maple syrup

Preparation:

Mix chia seeds and almond milk, refrigerate for at least 2 hours.

Layer chia pudding with mixed berries and sliced almonds.

Drizzle with maple syrup.

Nutritional Value:

Fiber: 7g

Protein: 5g

Calories: 220

Preparation Time: 5 minutes (plus chilling time)

15. Broccoli and Tomato Breakfast Muffins

Benefits:

Broccoli is easy on the stomach.

Tomatoes add flavor without acidity.

Muffins are convenient for on-the-go.

Ingredients:

2 cups broccoli, finely chopped

1 cup cherry tomatoes, diced

4 eggs

1/2 cup whole wheat flour

1/2 cup shredded cheese

Salt and pepper to taste

Preparation:

Mix broccoli, tomatoes, eggs, whole wheat flour, and shredded cheese.

Pour into muffin cups and bake at 375°F (190°C) for 20 minutes.

Nutritional Value:

Fiber: 5g

Protein: 10g

Calories: 250

Cooking Time: 20 minutes

CHAPTER 4: Lunch Recipes

1. Sweet Potato and Lentil Stew

Benefits:

Sweet potatoes provide vitamins and are gentle on the stomach.

Lentils offer protein and fiber for a satisfying and nutritious meal.

Ingredients:

2 sweet potatoes, peeled and diced

1 cup dry lentils, rinsed

1 onion, chopped

2 cloves garlic, minced

4 cups vegetable broth

1 teaspoon ground turmeric

Add Salt and pepper to taste better.

Preparation:

In a pot, sauté onions and garlic until fragrant.

Add sweet potatoes, lentils, vegetable broth, turmeric, salt, and pepper.

Simmer until lentils are tender, about 25-30 minutes.

Nutritional Value:

Fiber: 12g

Protein: 14g

Calories: 300

Cooking Time: 30 minutes

2. Mushroom and Spinach Quiche with Whole Wheat Crust

Benefits:

Mushrooms and spinach are gentle on the stomach.

Whole wheat crust adds fiber.

Ingredients:

1 whole wheat pie crust

2 cups mushrooms, sliced

2 cups fresh spinach

1 onion, diced

4 eggs

1 cup milk (dairy or plant-based)

Salt and pepper to taste

Preparation:

Sauté mushrooms and onions until softened.

In a bowl, whisk eggs and milk, season with salt and pepper.

Layer spinach, mushroom-onion mixture in the pie crust, pour the egg mixture over.

Bake at 375°F (190°C) for 35-40 minutes.

Nutritional Value:

Fiber: 7g

Protein: 10g

Calories: 320

Cooking Time: 40 minutes

3. Chickpea and Vegetable Stir-Fry with Brown Rice

Benefits:

Chickpeas provide protein and fiber.

Brown rice offers a gentle base for the stomach.

Ingredients:

1 cup cooked brown rice

1 can chickpeas, drained and rinsed

2 cups mixed vegetables (broccoli, bell peppers, snap peas)

2 tablespoons soy sauce

1 tablespoon sesame oil

1 teaspoon ginger, grated

Preparation:

Sauté mixed vegetables in sesame oil and ginger until tender.

Add chickpeas and cooked brown rice, stir-fry for a few minutes.

Drizzle with soy sauce and toss until well combined.

Nutritional Value:

Fiber: 8g

Protein: 12g

Calories: 350

Cooking Time: 20 minutes

4. Eggplant and Zucchini Lasagna

Benefits:

Eggplant and zucchini are low in acidity.

Plant-based lasagna for a comforting yet stomach-friendly meal.

Ingredients:

1 large eggplant, sliced

2 zucchinis, sliced

2 cups tomato sauce

1 cup ricotta cheese (or plant-based alternative)

1 cup spinach leaves

1/2 cup grated Parmesan cheese (or nutritional yeast)

1 teaspoon Italian seasoning

Preparation:

Grill or roast eggplant and zucchini slices until softened.

In a baking dish, layer tomato sauce, eggplant, zucchini, ricotta, spinach, and repeat.

Top with Parmesan cheese and Italian seasoning.

Bake at 375°F (190°C) for 30-35 minutes.

Nutritional Value:

Fiber: 9g

Protein: 15g

Calories: 380

Cooking Time: 35 minutes

5. Cauliflower and Chickpea Curry

Benefits:

Cauliflower and chickpeas provide fiber and protein.

Curry spices may have anti-inflammatory properties.

Ingredients:

1 cauliflower, cut into florets

1 can chickpeas, drained and rinsed

1 onion, diced

2 tomatoes, chopped

1 can coconut milk

2 tablespoons curry powder

1 teaspoon turmeric

Salt and pepper to taste

Preparation:

Sauté onions until translucent, add curry powder and turmeric.

Add cauliflower, chickpeas, tomatoes, and coconut milk.

Simmer until cauliflower is tender, about 20 minutes.

Nutritional Value:

Fiber: 10g

Protein: 12g

Calories: 320

Cooking Time: 20 minutes

6. Stuffed Bell Peppers with Quinoa and Black Beans

Benefits:

Bell peppers are gentle on the stomach.

Quinoa and black beans provide protein and fiber.

Ingredients:

4 bell peppers, halved

1 cup cooked quinoa

1 cup black beans, cooked

1 cup corn kernels (fresh or frozen)

1 cup salsa

1/2 cup shredded cheese (cheddar or plant-based)

Fresh cilantro, chopped

Preparation:

Preheat the oven to 375°F (190°C).

In a bowl, mix quinoa, black beans, corn, and salsa.

Stuff bell pepper halves with the mixture, top with shredded cheese.

Bake for 25-30 minutes until peppers are tender.

Nutritional Value:

Fiber: 8g

Protein: 10g

Calories: 330

Cooking Time: 30 minutes

7. Caprese Quinoa Salad

Benefits:

Quinoa provides protein and is easy on the stomach.

Tomatoes and basil offer vitamins and antioxidants.

Ingredients:

1 cup cooked quinoa

1 cup cherry tomatoes, halved

1 cup fresh mozzarella, diced

Fresh basil leaves, chopped

Balsamic vinaigrette dressing

Preparation:

In a bowl, combine quinoa, cherry tomatoes, mozzarella, and basil.

Drizzle with balsamic vinaigrette, toss gently.

Nutritional Value:

Fiber: 5g

Protein: 13g

Calories: 320

Preparation Time: 10 minutes

8. Lemon-Garlic Roasted Vegetable Wrap

Benefits:

Roasted vegetables are easy on the stomach.

Lemon and garlic add flavor without acidity.

Ingredients:

1 cup mixed vegetables (zucchini, bell peppers, cherry tomatoes)

1 tablespoon olive oil

1 teaspoon lemon zest

1 clove garlic, minced

1 whole grain tortilla

Hummus for spreading

Preparation:

Toss mixed vegetables with olive oil, lemon zest, and minced garlic.

Roast in the oven at 400°F (200°C) for 20 minutes.

Spread hummus on a whole grain tortilla, add roasted vegetables, and wrap.

Nutritional Value:

Fiber: 7g

Protein: 8g

Calories: 280

Cooking Time: 20 minutes

9. Cucumber and Avocado Sushi Bowl

Benefits:

Cucumber and avocado are easy on the stomach.

Sushi flavors without the need for raw fish.

Ingredients:

2 cups cooked sushi rice

1 cucumber, sliced

1 avocado, diced

Nori seaweed, shredded

Soy sauce for drizzling

Pickled ginger and wasabi (optional)

Preparation:

In a bowl, layer cooked sushi rice, cucumber, and avocado.

Top with shredded nori seaweed.

Drizzle with soy sauce and add pickled ginger and wasabi if desired.

Nutritional Value:

Fiber: 6g

Protein: 5g

Calories: 290

Preparation Time: 15 minutes

10. Broccoli and Almond Stir-Fry with Quinoa

Benefits:

Broccoli and almonds provide vitamins and minerals.

Quinoa offers protein and is easy on the stomach.

Ingredients:

1 cup cooked quinoa

2 cups broccoli florets

1/4 cup almonds, sliced

2 tablespoons soy sauce

1 tablespoon sesame oil

1 teaspoon honey

1 clove garlic, minced

Preparation:

Sauté broccoli in sesame oil until slightly tender.

Add almonds, soy sauce, honey, and minced garlic.

Stir-fry until broccoli is crisp-tender.

Serve over cooked quinoa.

Nutritional Value:

Fiber: 7g

Protein: 9g

Calories: 310

Cooking Time: 15 minutes

11. Tomato and White Bean Soup

Benefits:

Tomatoes offer vitamins and antioxidants.

White beans provide protein and fiber.

Ingredients:

2 cups canned white beans, drained and rinsed

1 can diced tomatoes

1 onion, chopped

2 carrots, sliced

2 cups vegetable broth

1 teaspoon dried basil

Salt and pepper to taste cool

Preparation:

Sauté onions and carrots until softened.

Add white beans, diced tomatoes, vegetable broth, basil, salt, and pepper.

Simmer for 20-25 minutes.

Nutritional Value:

Fiber: 8g

Protein: 10g

Calories: 280

Cooking Time: 25 minutes

12. Greek Chickpea Salad Wrap

Benefits:

Chickpeas offer protein and fiber.

Greek flavors without the heaviness of meat.

Ingredients:

1 can chickpeas, drained and rinsed

1 cucumber, diced

1 tomato, diced

1/4 cup red onion, finely chopped

Feta cheese, crumbled

Hummus for spreading

Whole grain tortilla

Preparation:

In a bowl, mix chickpeas, cucumber, tomato, red onion, and feta.

Spread hummus on a whole grain tortilla, add the chickpea mixture, and wrap.

Nutritional Value:

Fiber: 7g

Protein: 10g

Calories: 310

Preparation Time: 10 minutes

13. Lentil and Vegetable Buddha Bowl

Benefits:

Lentils provide protein and fiber.

Colorful vegetables for a variety of nutrients.

Ingredients:

1 cup cooked lentils

1 cup roasted sweet potatoes

1 cup sautéed kale

1/2 cup shredded purple cabbage

Avocado slices

Tahini dressing

Preparation:

Arrange cooked lentils, roasted sweet potatoes, sautéed kale, shredded cabbage, and avocado in a bowl.

Drizzle with tahini dressing.

Nutritional Value:

Fiber: 10g

Protein: 15g

Calories: 340

Preparation Time: 20 minutes

Benefits:

Tofu provides plant-based protein.

Ginger may have anti-inflammatory properties.

Ingredients:

1 cup firm tofu, cubed

2 cups mixed vegetables (broccoli, bell peppers, snap peas)

1 cup cooked brown rice

2 tablespoons miso paste

1 tablespoon soy sauce

1 teaspoon fresh ginger, grated

Preparation:

Sauté tofu until golden.

Add mixed vegetables, cooked brown rice, miso paste, soy sauce, and ginger.

Stir-fry until vegetables are tender.

Nutritional Value:

Fiber: 8g

Protein: 12g

Calories: 330

Cooking Time: 15 minutes

15. Spaghetti Squash Primavera

Benefits:

Spaghetti squash is a light alternative to pasta.

Colorful vegetables for added nutrients.

Ingredients:

1 spaghetti squash, halved and seeded

1 cup cherry tomatoes, halved

1 zucchini, diced

1 bell pepper, sliced

2 cloves garlic, minced

2 tablespoons olive oil

Fresh basil, chopped

Preparation:

Roast spaghetti squash in the oven at 375°F (190°C) for 40 minutes.

Sauté cherry tomatoes, zucchini, bell pepper, and garlic in olive oil.

Scrape the spaghetti squash strands into a bowl, top with sautéed vegetables, and garnish with fresh basil.

Nutritional Value:

Fiber: 9g

Protein: 5g

Calories: 250

Cooking Time: 40 minutes

CHAPTER 5: Salads for Gut Health

1. Quinoa and Chickpea Mediterranean Salad

Benefits:

Quinoa provides complete protein.

Chickpeas offer fiber and protein.

Mediterranean ingredients for anti-inflammatory effects.

Ingredients:

1 cup cooked quinoa

1 cup canned chickpeas, drained and rinsed

1 cucumber, diced

1 cup cherry tomatoes, halved

1/4 cup red onion, finely chopped

Feta cheese, crumbled (optional)

Kalamata olives, sliced

Olive oil and lemon juice for dressing

Preparation:

Combine quinoa, chickpeas, cucumber, tomatoes, red onion, feta, and olives.

Drizzle with olive oil and lemon juice, toss gently.

Nutritional Value:

Fiber: 8g

Protein: 10g

Calories: 300

Preparation Time: 15 minutes

2. Spinach and Strawberry Salad with Almond Vinaigrette

Benefits:

Spinach provides vitamins and minerals.

Strawberries offer antioxidants.

Almonds add healthy fats.

Ingredients:

2 cups fresh spinach leaves

1 cup strawberries, sliced

1/4 cup almonds, sliced

Feta cheese, crumbled (optional)

2 tablespoons balsamic vinaigrette

Preparation:

In a bowl, combine spinach, strawberries, almonds, and feta.

Drizzle with balsamic vinaigrette, toss gently.

Nutritional Value:

Fiber: 6g

Protein: 5g

Calories: 250

Preparation Time: 10 minutes

3. Cauliflower and Broccoli Detox Salad

Benefits:

Cauliflower and broccoli aid digestion.

Detoxifying ingredients for overall wellness.

Ingredients:

2 cups cauliflower florets, finely chopped

2 cups broccoli florets, finely chopped

1/2 cup carrots, shredded

1/4 cup sunflower seeds

1/4 cup raisins

Greek yogurt and lemon dressing

Preparation:

Mix cauliflower, broccoli, carrots, sunflower seeds, and raisins.

Toss with Greek yogurt and lemon dressing.

Nutritional Value:

Fiber: 7g

Protein: 6g

Calories: 220

Preparation Time: 15 minutes

4. Avocado and Black Bean Fiesta Salad

Benefits:

Avocado provides healthy fats.

Black beans offer protein and fiber.

Colorful veggies for a nutrient-rich salad.

Ingredients:

1 avocado, diced

1 cup canned black beans, drained and rinsed

1 cup corn kernels (fresh or frozen)

1 bell pepper, diced

1/4 cup red onion, finely chopped

Fresh cilantro, chopped

Lime vinaigrette dressing

Preparation:

Combine avocado, black beans, corn, bell pepper, red onion, and cilantro.

Drizzle with lime vinaigrette, toss gently.

Nutritional Value:

Fiber: 9g

Protein: 8g

Calories: 320

Preparation Time: 15 minutes

5. Mango and Quinoa Summer Salad

Benefits:

Mango provides vitamins A and C.

Quinoa offers protein and fiber.

Light and refreshing for a summer salad.

Ingredients:

1 cup cooked quinoa

1 mango, diced

1 cucumber, diced

1/4 cup red bell pepper, diced

Fresh mint leaves, chopped

Lime juice and honey dressing

Preparation:

Mix quinoa, mango, cucumber, red bell pepper, and mint.

Drizzle with lime juice and honey dressing, toss gently

.

Nutritional Value:

Fiber: 7g

Protein: 6g

Calories: 280

Preparation Time: 10 minutes

6. Greek Salad with Tofu Feta

Benefits:

Tofu provides plant-based protein.

Greek ingredients for a flavorful and satisfying salad.

Ingredients:

2 cups cherry tomatoes, halved

1 cucumber, diced

1/2 cup red onion, thinly sliced

1/2 cup Kalamata olives, sliced

Tofu feta (tofu marinated in olive oil, lemon juice, oregano)

Preparation:

Combine cherry tomatoes, cucumber, red onion, and Kalamata olives.

Add tofu feta on top.

Nutritional Value:

Fiber: 6g

Protein: 8g

Calories: 250

Preparation Time: 15 minutes

7. Roasted Beet and Lentil Salad

Benefits:

Beets provide antioxidants and aid digestion.

Lentils offer protein and fiber.

Warm salad option for added comfort.

Ingredients:

2 medium beets, roasted and sliced

1 cup cooked lentils

1 cup arugula

1/4 cup goat cheese, crumbled

Balsamic vinaigrette dressing

Preparation:

Roast beets, let them cool, and slice.

Mix beets, lentils, arugula, and goat cheese.

Drizzle with balsamic vinaigrette, toss gently.

Nutritional Value:

Fiber: 8g

Protein: 9g

Calories: 290

Preparation Time: 25 minutes

8. Pear and Walnut Spinach Salad

Benefits:

Pears offer fiber and natural sweetness.

Walnuts provide omega-3 fatty acids.

Spinach is gentle on the stomach.

Ingredients:

2 cups fresh spinach leaves

1 pear, sliced

1/4 cup walnuts, chopped

1/4 cup feta cheese, crumbled

Honey Dijon mustard dressing

Preparation:

Combine spinach, pear, walnuts, and feta.

Drizzle with honey Dijon mustard dressing, toss gently.

Nutritional Value:

Fiber: 6g

Protein: 7g

Calories: 260

Preparation Time: 10 minutes

9. Tomato and Basil Caprese Salad

Benefits:

Tomatoes and basil offer vitamins and antioxidants.

Mozzarella provides protein and creaminess.

Light and refreshing classic salad.

Ingredients:

1 cup cherry tomatoes, halved

1 cup fresh mozzarella, diced

Fresh basil leaves

Balsamic glaze for drizzling

Preparation:

Arrange cherry tomatoes, mozzarella, and fresh basil on a plate.

Drizzle with balsamic glaze.

Nutritional Value:

Fiber: 2g

Protein: 14g

Calories: 230

Preparation Time: 5 minutes

10. Arugula and Orange Citrus Salad

Benefits:

Arugula provides a peppery flavor.

Oranges offer vitamin C and natural sweetness.

Citrus dressing for a zesty kick.

Ingredients:

2 cups arugula

2 oranges, peeled and segmented

1/4 cup red onion, thinly sliced

1/4 cup pistachios, chopped

Citrus dressing (orange juice, olive oil, Dijon mustard)

Preparation:

Toss arugula, orange segments, red onion, and pistachios.

Drizzle with citrus dressing, toss gently.

Nutritional Value:

Fiber: 5g

Protein: 4g

Calories: 240

Preparation Time: 10 minutes

CHAPTER 6: Soothing Soups and Stews

1. Healing Turmeric and Ginger Carrot Soup

Benefits:

Turmeric and ginger may have anti-inflammatory properties.

Carrots are gentle on the stomach and rich in vitamins.

Ingredients:

4 cups carrots, chopped

1 onion, diced

2 tablespoons fresh ginger, grated

1 tablespoon turmeric powder

4 cups vegetable broth

Salt and pepper to taste

Coconut milk for creaminess (optional)

Preparation:

Sauté onions and ginger until fragrant.

Add carrots, turmeric, vegetable broth, salt, and pepper.

Simmer until carrots are tender, then blend until smooth.

Stir in coconut milk if desired.

Nutritional Value:

Fiber: 6g

Protein: 3g

Calories: 180

Cooking Time: 30 minutes

2. Nourishing Spinach and Lentil Soup

Benefits:

Spinach is easy on the stomach and rich in nutrients.

Lentils provide protein and fiber.

Ingredients:

1 cup dry lentils, rinsed

4 cups fresh spinach leaves

1 onion, chopped

2 carrots, sliced

2 cloves garlic, minced

6 cups vegetable broth

1 teaspoon cumin

Salt and pepper to taste

Preparation:

Sauté onions and garlic until softened.

Add lentils, carrots, cumin, vegetable broth, salt, and pepper.

Simmer until lentils are cooked, then stir in fresh spinach.

Nutritional Value:

Fiber: 10g

Protein: 15g

Calories: 280

Cooking Time: 40 minutes

3. Mild Butternut Squash and Apple Soup

Benefits:

Butternut squash is easy on the stomach.

Apples add natural sweetness and vitamins.

Ingredients:

1 medium butternut squash, peeled and diced

2 apples, peeled and chopped

1 onion, diced

4 cups vegetable broth

1 teaspoon cinnamon

1/2 teaspoon nutmeg

Salt and pepper to taste

Preparation:

Sauté onions until translucent.

Add butternut squash, apples, vegetable broth, cinnamon, nutmeg, salt, and pepper.

Simmer until squash is tender, then blend until smooth.

Nutritional Value:

Fiber: 8g

Protein: 2g

Calories: 200

Cooking Time: 35 minutes

4. Zesty Quinoa and Kale Soup

Benefits:

Quinoa provides protein and is easy to digest.

Kale is rich in vitamins and minerals.

Ingredients:

1 cup cooked quinoa

4 cups kale, chopped

1 onion, diced

2 carrots, sliced

2 cloves garlic, minced

6 cups vegetable broth

1 lemon, juiced

Salt and pepper to taste

Preparation:

Sauté onions and garlic until fragrant.

Add carrots, kale, vegetable broth, salt, and pepper.

Simmer until vegetables are tender, and then stir in cooked quinoa.

Finish with fresh lemon juice before serving.

Nutritional Value:

Fiber: 7g

Protein: 10g

Calories: 300

Cooking Time: 30 minutes

5. Comforting Chickpea and Rice Soup

Benefits:

Chickpeas offer protein and fiber.

Rice provides a gentle base for the stomach.

Ingredients:

1 can chickpeas, drained and rinsed

1 cup cooked rice

1 onion, chopped

2 carrots, sliced

2 celery stalks, chopped

2 cloves garlic, minced

6 cups vegetable broth

1 teaspoon thyme

Salt and pepper to taste

Preparation:

Sauté onions and garlic until softened.

Add carrots, celery, chickpeas, vegetable broth, thyme, salt, and pepper.

Simmer until vegetables are tender, and then stir in cooked rice.

Nutritional Value:

Fiber: 8g

Protein: 10g

Calories: 320

Cooking Time: 35 minutes

6. Soothing Potato and Leek Soup

Benefits:

Potatoes are easy on the stomach and provide energy.

Leeks add a mild onion flavor without the acidity.

Ingredients:

3 potatoes, peeled and diced

2 leeks, sliced

1 onion, diced

4 cups vegetable broth

1 cup unsweetened almond milk

2 tablespoons olive oil

Salt and pepper to taste

Preparation:

Sauté leeks and onions in olive oil until softened.

Add potatoes, vegetable broth, almond milk, salt, and pepper.

Simmer until potatoes are tender, then blend until smooth.

Nutritional Value:

Fiber: 6g

Protein: 4g

Calories: 220

Cooking Time: 25 minutes

7. Refreshing Cucumber and Avocado Gazpacho

Benefits:

Cucumbers and avocados are gentle on the stomach.

Cold gazpacho for a soothing and hydrating option.

Ingredients:

2 cucumbers, peeled and chopped

1 avocado, diced

1 bell pepper, diced

2 cloves garlic, minced

4 cups vegetable broth

1/4 cup fresh cilantro, chopped

1 lime, juiced

Salt and pepper to taste better

Preparation:

In a blender, combine cucumbers, avocado, bell pepper, garlic, vegetable broth, cilantro, lime juice, salt, and pepper.

Blend until smooth.

Chill in the refrigerator before serving.

Nutritional Value:

Fiber: 7g

Protein: 4g

Calories: 250

Preparation Time: 15 minutes

8. Tomato and Basil Quinoa Soup

Benefits:

Quinoa provides protein and is easy to digest.

Tomatoes and basil offer vitamins and antioxidants.

Ingredients:

1 cup cooked quinoa

1 can diced tomatoes

1 onion, diced

2 carrots, sliced

2 cloves garlic, minced

6 cups vegetable broth

Fresh basil leaves, chopped

Salt and pepper to taste good.

Preparation:

Sauté onions and garlic until fragrant.

Add carrots, diced tomatoes, vegetable broth, salt, and pepper.

Simmer until carrots are tender, then stir in cooked quinoa.

Garnish with fresh basil before serving.

Nutritional Value:

Fiber: 9g

Protein: 7g

Calories: 270

Cooking Time: 30 minutes

9. Broccoli and Almond Creamy Soup

Benefits:

Broccoli is easy on the stomach and rich in vitamins.

Almonds add creaminess without dairy.

Ingredients:

2 cups broccoli florets

1/2 cup almonds, soaked

1 onion, chopped

2 cloves garlic, minced

4 cups vegetable broth

1 cup unsweetened almond milk

2 tablespoons nutritional yeast

Salt and pepper to taste

Preparation:

Sauté onions and garlic until softened.

Add broccoli, soaked almonds, vegetable broth, almond milk, nutritional yeast, salt, and pepper.

Simmer until broccoli is tender, then blend until creamy.

Nutritional Value:

Fiber: 8g

Protein: 10g

Calories: 290

Cooking Time: 25 minutes

10. Mushroom and Brown Rice Congee

Benefits:

Mushrooms are easy to digest and provide a savory flavor.

Brown rice offers a gentle base for the stomach.

Ingredients:

1 cup brown rice, uncooked

1 cup mushrooms, sliced

1 inch ginger, grated

6 cups vegetable broth

2 tablespoons soy sauce

Green onions for garnish

Sesame oil for drizzling

Preparation:

Rinse brown rice and cook it with vegetable broth until soft and porridge-like.

In a separate pan, sauté mushrooms and ginger until tender.

Stir sautéed mushrooms into the rice congee.

Season with soy sauce, garnish with green onions, and drizzle with sesame oil.

Nutritional Value:

Fiber: 6g

Protein: 9g

Calories: 260

Cooking Time: 40 minutes

CHAPTER 7: Beverages for Stomach Comfort

1. Soothing Ginger and Mint Tea

Benefits:

Ginger may help alleviate nausea and inflammation.

Mint provides a refreshing and soothing flavor.

Ingredients:

1-inch fresh ginger, sliced

Handful of fresh mint leaves

4 cups hot water

Optional: Lemon wedges and honey for taste

Preparation:

Place ginger slices and mint leaves in a teapot.

Pour hot water over them and let steep for 5-7 minutes.

Strain the tea and add lemon wedges or honey if desired.

Nutritional Value:

Ginger may aid digestion.

Mint can help soothe the stomach.

Calories: Negligible

Preparation Time: 10 minutes

2. Calming Chamomile and Lavender Infusion

Benefits:

Chamomile has anti-inflammatory properties.

Lavender may help reduce stress and promote relaxation.

Ingredients:

2 chamomile tea bags

1 tablespoon dried lavender flowers

4 cups hot water

Optional: A drizzle of honey

Preparation:

Steep chamomile tea bags and dried lavender in hot water for 5-8 minutes.

Remove tea bags and strain the infusion.

Add honey if desired.

Nutritional Value:

Chamomile may aid in digestion and soothe the stomach.

Lavender may promote relaxation.

Calories: Negligible

Preparation Time: 10 minutes

3. Balancing Almond and Banana Smoothie

Benefits:

Almonds provide healthy fats and protein.

Banana is a gentle and easily digestible fruit.

Ingredients:

1 ripe banana

1 cup almond milk (unsweetened)

1 tablespoon almond butter

1/2 teaspoon vanilla extract

Ice cubes (optional)

Preparation:

Blend banana, almond milk, almond butter, and vanilla extract until smooth.

Add ice cubes if a colder consistency is desired.

Nutritional Value:

Almonds provide protein and healthy fats.

Banana is easy on the stomach.

Calories: 250

Preparation Time: 5 minutes

4. Cucumber and Aloe Vera Cooler

Benefits:

Cucumber is hydrating and may help reduce acidity.

Aloe vera may have soothing properties.

Ingredients:

1 cucumber, sliced

2 tablespoons fresh aloe vera gel

4 cups cold water

Mint leaves for garnish

Ice cubes

Preparation:

Blend cucumber and aloe vera with cold water until well combined.

Strain the mixture and pour over ice.

Garnish with mint leaves.

Nutritional Value:

Cucumber provides hydration.

Aloe vera may have soothing effects.

Calories: Negligible

Preparation Time: 10 minutes

5. Papaya and Pineapple Digestive Elixir

Benefits:

Papaya contains enzymes that aid digestion.

Pineapple provides bromelain, known for its anti-inflammatory properties.

Ingredients:

1 cup fresh papaya, diced

1 cup fresh pineapple, diced

1 tablespoon fresh lime juice

2 cups cold water

Ice cubes

Preparation:

Blend papaya, pineapple, lime juice, and cold water until smooth.

Pour over ice and serve immediately.

Nutritional Value:

Papaya aids digestion.

Pineapple may have anti-inflammatory effects.

Calories: 150

Preparation Time: 5 minutes

6. Chia Seed and Berry Hydration Drink

Benefits:

Chia seeds provide omega-3 fatty acids and fiber.

Berries are rich in antioxidants.

Ingredients:

2 tablespoons chia seeds

1 cup mixed berries (strawberries, blueberries, raspberries)

4 cups cold water

1 tablespoon maple syrup (optional)

Preparation:

Mix chia seeds with cold water and let sit for 10 minutes.

Blend the mixed berries with the chia gel until smooth.

Strain the mixture if desired and sweeten with maple syrup.

Nutritional Value:

Chia seeds offer omega-3 fatty acids and fiber.

Berries provide antioxidants.

Calories: 100

Preparation Time: 15 minutes

7. Anti-Inflammatory Golden Milk

Benefits:

Turmeric in golden milk has anti-inflammatory properties.

Black pepper enhances the absorption of curcumin in turmeric.

Ingredients:

1 cup almond milk (unsweetened)

1 teaspoon ground turmeric

1/2 teaspoon ground cinnamon

1/4 teaspoon ground ginger

Pinch of black pepper

1 tablespoon honey (optional)

Preparation:

Heat almond milk in a saucepan over medium heat.

Add turmeric, cinnamon, ginger, and black pepper.

Whisk continuously until warm, but not boiling.

Sweeten with honey if desired.

Nutritional Value:

Turmeric has anti-inflammatory properties.

Almond milk provides calcium and vitamin D.

Calories: 70

Preparation Time: 5 minutes

8. Raspberry and Lemon Balm Iced Tea

Benefits:

Raspberry may provide antioxidants.

Lemon balm is known for its calming effects.

Ingredients:

1 cup fresh raspberries

1/4 cup fresh lemon balm leaves

2 black tea bags

4 cups hot water

2 tablespoons honey (optional)

Ice cubes

Preparation:

Steep black tea bags, raspberries, and lemon balm in hot water for 5-7 minutes.

Strain the tea and sweeten with honey if desired.

Chill in the refrigerator and serve over ice.

Nutritional Value:

Raspberries offer antioxidants.

Lemon balm may have calming effects.

Calories: 50

Preparation Time: 10 minutes

9. Peppermint and Fennel Seed Infusion

Benefits:

Peppermint is known for its soothing properties.

Fennel seeds may help relieve digestive discomfort.

Ingredients:

1 tablespoon dried peppermint leaves

1 tablespoon fennel seeds

4 cups hot water

Lemon slices for garnish

Honey for sweetness (optional)

Preparation:

Steep dried peppermint leaves and fennel seeds in hot water for 7-10 minutes.

Strain the infusion and garnish with lemon slices.

Sweeten with honey if desired.

Nutritional Value:

Peppermint may soothe digestive issues.

Fennel seeds may help relieve bloating.

Calories: Negligible

Preparation Time: 10 minutes

10. Probiotic-rich Coconut Water Kefir

Benefits:

Coconut water is hydrating.

Kefir contains probiotics for gut health.

Ingredients:

2 cups coconut water

2 tablespoons kefir grains

1 tablespoon maple syrup (optional)

Preparation:

Combine coconut water and kefir grains in a glass jar.

Cover the jar with a cloth and secure with a rubber band.

Allow it to ferment at room temperature for 24-48 hours.

Strain the kefir grains and sweeten with maple syrup if desired.

Nutritional Value:

Coconut water provides hydration.

Kefir offers probiotics for gut health.

Calories: 50

Fermentation Time: 24-48 hours

CHAPTER 8: Sweet Dessert for the soul

1. Banana and Almond Butter Rice Cake Delight

Benefits:

Bananas are gentle on the stomach and provide natural sweetness.

Almond butter offers healthy fats and protein.

Ingredients:

2 rice cakes

2 ripe bananas, sliced

4 tablespoons almond butter

Cinnamon for sprinkling

Preparation:

Spread almond butter on rice cakes.

Top with banana slices and sprinkle with cinnamon.

Nutritional Value:

Fiber: 4g

Protein: 6g

Calories: 300

Preparation Time: 5 minutes

2. Chia Seed Pudding with Mixed Berries

Benefits:

Chia seeds provide omega-3 fatty acids and fiber.

Berries are rich in antioxidants.

Ingredients:

3 tablespoons chia seeds

1 cup almond milk (unsweetened)

1 teaspoon vanilla extract

Mixed berries for topping

Preparation:

Mix chia seeds, almond milk, and vanilla extract in a bowl.

Refrigerate for at least 4 hours or overnight until it thickens.

Top with mixed berries before serving.

Nutritional Value:

Fiber: 10g

Protein: 5g

Calories: 220

Preparation Time: 5 minutes (plus chilling time)

3. Avocado Chocolate Mousse

Benefits:

Avocado provides healthy fats and a creamy texture.

Cocoa powder adds rich chocolate flavor.

Ingredients:

2 ripe avocados

1/4 cup cocoa powder

1/4 cup maple syrup

1 teaspoon vanilla extract

Preparation:

Blend avocados, cocoa powder, maple syrup, and vanilla extract until smooth.

Chill in the refrigerator for at least 30 minutes before serving.

Nutritional Value:

Fiber: 7g

Protein: 4g

Calories: 250

Preparation Time: 10 minutes

4. Coconut Yogurt Parfait with Granola

Benefits:

Coconut yogurt is a dairy-free option for gut health.

Granola provides crunch and fiber.

Ingredients:

1 cup coconut yogurt

1/2 cup granola

Fresh fruit for topping (e.g., berries, kiwi)

Preparation:

Layer coconut yogurt, granola, and fresh fruit in a glass or bowl.

Repeat the layers until the container is filled.

Nutritional Value:

Fiber: 6g

Protein: 7g

Calories: 320

Preparation Time: 5 minutes

5. Pumpkin and Oat Muffins

Benefits:

Pumpkin is easy on the stomach and provides vitamins.

Oats offer fiber and are gentle on digestion.

Ingredients:

1 cup canned pumpkin

1 cup rolled oats

1/4 cup maple syrup

1 teaspoon baking powder

1/2 teaspoon cinnamon

Preparation:

Mix pumpkin, rolled oats, maple syrup, baking powder, and cinnamon in a bowl.

Scoop into muffin cups and bake at 350°F (175°C) for 20 minutes.

Nutritional Value:

Fiber: 5g

Protein: 3g

Calories: 180

Cooking Time: 20 minutes

6. Almond and Berry Frozen Yogurt Popsicles

Benefits:

Almonds provide healthy fats and protein.

Berries offer antioxidants and natural sweetness.

Ingredients:

1 cup almond milk yogurt

1/2 cup mixed berries (e.g., strawberries, blueberries)

2 tablespoons almond slices

Preparation:

Mix almond milk yogurt and mixed berries.

Spoon the mixture into popsicle molds and sprinkle with almond slices.

Freeze for at least 4 hours.

Nutritional Value:

Fiber: 3g

Protein: 4g

Calories: 150

Freezing Time: 4 hours

7. Mango and Coconut Chia Seed Sorbet

Benefits:

Mango provides vitamins and natural sweetness.

Coconut milk adds creaminess.

Ingredients:

2 cups frozen mango chunks

1/2 cup coconut milk

2 tablespoons chia seeds

Preparation:

Blend frozen mango and coconut milk until smooth.

Stir in chia seeds and freeze for at least 2 hours.

Nutritional Value:

Fiber: 6g

Protein: 4g

Calories: 220

Freezing Time: 2 hours

8. Walnut and Date Energy Balls

Benefits:

Walnuts offer omega-3 fatty acids.

Dates provide natural sweetness and fiber.

Ingredients:

1 cup walnuts

1 cup dates, pitted

1/2 cup shredded coconut

1 teaspoon vanilla extract

Preparation:

Blend walnuts, dates, shredded coconut, and vanilla extract in a food processor.

Roll the mixture into small balls and refrigerate for 1 hour.

Nutritional Value:

Fiber: 4g

Protein: 5g

Calories: 250

Chilling Time: 1 hour

9. Blueberry and Almond Oat Bars

Benefits:

Blueberries provide antioxidants and natural sweetness.

Almonds offer healthy fats and protein.

Ingredients:

2 cups rolled oats

1 cup almond butter

1/2 cup maple syrup

1 cup blueberries

Preparation:

Mix rolled oats, almond butter, and maple syrup in a bowl.

Fold in blueberries and press the mixture into a baking dish.

Bake at 350°F (175°C) for 25 minutes.

Nutritional Value:

Fiber: 6g

Protein: 8g

Calories: 320

Baking Time: 25 minutes

10. Cinnamon and Apple Quinoa Pudding

Benefits:

Apples are easy on the stomach and provide vitamins.

Quinoa offers protein and is gentle on digestion.

Ingredients:

1 cup cooked quinoa

1 apple, diced

2 tablespoons maple syrup

1/2 teaspoon cinnamon

1/4 cup chopped walnuts

Preparation:

Mix cooked quinoa, diced apple, maple syrup, and cinnamon.

Top with chopped walnuts before serving.

Nutritional Value:

Fiber: 5g

Protein: 6g

Calories: 280

Preparation Time: 5 minutes

CONCLUSION

This Stomach Ulcer Cookbook for Vegetarians offers a holistic approach to healing and maintaining digestive wellness through a plant-based diet. By adopting nutrient-rich, easily digestible, and anti-inflammatory foods, this cookbook aims to provide relief and support for individuals dealing with stomach ulcers. The recipes curated here not only focus on soothing and nourishing the digestive system but also celebrate the diverse flavors and textures of vegetarian ingredients.

Understanding the importance of key nutrients, this cookbook incorporates a variety of plant-based sources that contribute to the healing process. From fiber-rich grains and legumes to antioxidant-packed fruits and vegetables, each recipe is thoughtfully crafted to promote gastric health while ensuring a delightful culinary experience. The inclusion of specific foods known for their digestive benefits, such as ginger, turmeric, and probiotic-rich options, reflects a commitment to addressing the unique needs of individuals managing stomach ulcers.

Moreover, the cookbook provides a wide array of options, including breakfasts, lunches, soups, beverages, and desserts, ensuring a well-rounded and enjoyable vegetarian gastronomic journey. It is my sincere hope that adopting this diet will not only aids in the physical recovery from stomach ulcers but also fosters a positive relationship with food and nourishment.

THANK YOU

Thank you for reading this cookbook till the end let this cookbook be your ally, your guide, and your source of inspiration. May each bite be a step toward comfort, and may the joy of eating return without the shadow of pain. Your journey to stomach ulcer management starts here, a journey not just of healing but of rediscovery and newfound resilience.

Happy Cooking!

7-WEEKS MEAL PLAN JOURNAL

WEEK 1:

WEEKLY MEAL PLANNER

START DATE ___________________ END DATE ___________________

MONDAY

SATURDAY

TUESDAY

SUNDAY

WEDNESDAY

SHOPPING LIST

- ○ ___________________
- ○ ___________________
- ○ ___________________
- ○ ___________________
- ○ ___________________
- ○ ___________________
- ○ ___________________

THURSDAY

COMMENT

FRIDAY

WEEK 2:

WEEKLY MEAL PLANNER

START DATE ______________________   END DATE ______________________

MONDAY

SATURDAY

TUESDAY

SUNDAY

WEDNESDAY

SHOPPING LIST

THURSDAY

COMMENT

FRIDAY

WEEK 3:

WEEKLY MEAL PLANNER

START DATE ______________________   END DATE ______________________

MONDAY

SATURDAY

TUESDAY

SUNDAY

WEDNESDAY

SHOPPING LIST

THURSDAY

COMMENT

FRIDAY

WEEK 4:

WEEKLY MEAL PLANNER

START DATE _______________   END DATE _______________

MONDAY

SATURDAY

TUESDAY

SUNDAY

WEDNESDAY

SHOPPING LIST
- ___________________
- ___________________
- ___________________
- ___________________
- ___________________
- ___________________
- ___________________

THURSDAY

COMMENT

FRIDAY

WEEK 5:

WEEKLY MEAL PLANNER

START DATE ___________________   END DATE ___________________

MONDAY

TUESDAY

WEDNESDAY

THURSDAY

FRIDAY

SATURDAY

SUNDAY

SHOPPING LIST

- ○ _______________
- ○ _______________
- ○ _______________
- ○ _______________
- ○ _______________
- ○ _______________
- ○ _______________

COMMENT

WEEK 6:

WEEKLY MEAL PLANNER

START DATE ______________________ END DATE ______________________

MONDAY

TUESDAY

WEDNESDAY

THURSDAY

FRIDAY

SATURDAY

SUNDAY

SHOPPING LIST

COMMENT

WEEK 7:

WEEKLY MEAL PLANNER

START DATE .... END DATE ....

MONDAY

SATURDAY

TUESDAY

SUNDAY

WEDNESDAY

SHOPPING LIST

THURSDAY

COMMENT

FRIDAY